THE NEWEST TYPE 2 DIABETIC COOKBOOK FOR BEGINNERS

2000+ Days Of Healthy And Delicious low-carb, low-suag and low-fat recipes for type 2 diabetes and prediabetes, with a 31-day meal plan

Angelo Melvin

Table of Contents

- CHAPTER ONE 4
- Understanding Type 2 Diabetes 4
- What is Type 2 Diabetes: Causes, Symptoms, and Risk Factors. 4
- Causes 5
- Symptoms 6
- Risk Factors 7
- The Importance of Diet and Lifestyle in Managing Type 2 Diabetes 8
- Dietary Strategies 8
- Physical Activity 10
- Stress Management and Sleep 10
- Monitoring and Medication 11
- Key Principles of a Diabetes-Friendly Diet for Beginners 11
- CHAPTER TWO 14
- Getting Started with Type 2 Diabetes Cooking 14
- Introduction to Diabetes-Friendly Ingredients and Substitutions 14
- Essential Kitchen Tools and Equipment for Beginner Cooks 18
- Tips for Grocery Shopping and Meal Planning for Diabetes Management 21
- CHAPTER THREE 24

- Breakfasts to Start Your Day Right 24
- Quick and Healthy Breakfast Ideas for Busy Mornings 24
- High-Fiber Breakfasts to Regulate Blood Sugar Levels 28
- Protein-Packed Breakfasts to Keep You Full and Energized 31

CHAPTER FOUR 35
- Simple and Satisfying Lunches 35
- Easy Salad and Wrap Recipes for Balanced Lunches 35
- Flavorful Soup and Sandwich Combos for Comforting Meals..39

CHAPTER FIVE 51
- Flavorful Dinners in a Flash 51
- One-Pot Dinners for Minimal Cleanup and Maximum Flavor..51
- Quick and Easy Stir-Fries for Busy Evenings............................55
- Comforting Casseroles and Skillet Meals for Weeknight Dinners 59

CHAPTER SEVEN 65
- Delicious Diabetic-Friendly Desserts 65
- Lower-Sugar Dessert Recipes for Satisfying Sweet Cravings ...65
- Fruit-Based Desserts That Are Naturally Sweet and Nutritious 69
- Indulgent Treats Made Healthier with Smart Ingredient Swaps 72

CHAPTER EIGHT..76

Side Dishes That Complement Any Meal 76

Simple and Delicious Vegetable Side Dishes 76

Whole Grain and Legume-Based Sides for Balanced Nutrition 79

CHAPTER NINE 87

Eating Out and Socializing with Diabetes 87

Strategies for Making Healthy Choices When Dining Out 87

Tips for Navigating Social Events and Special Occasions 88

CHAPTER TEN 91

Meal Planning and Preparation Made Easy 91

Practical Tips for Meal Planning and Grocery Shopping 91

Batch Cooking and Freezing Meals for Convenience 93

Strategies for Portion Control and Balanced Eating 95

CHAPTER 12 97

31 DAY MEAL PLAN 97

THE END 110

COPYRIGHT © 2023

All rights reserved. No part of this publication may be reproduced, distributed, or transmitted in any form or by any means, including photocopying, recording, or other electronic or mechanical methods, without the prior written permission of the publisher, except in the case of brief quotations embodied in critical reviews and certain other noncommercial uses permitted by copyright law.

CHAPTER ONE

Understanding Type 2 Diabetes

What is Type 2 Diabetes: Causes, Symptoms, and Risk Factors

Type 2 diabetes is a chronic metabolic disorder characterized by high levels of blood sugar (glucose) resulting from the body's ineffective use of insulin. Insulin is a hormone produced by the pancreas that helps regulate blood sugar levels by facilitating the uptake of glucose into cells for energy production. In individuals with type 2 diabetes, the body either doesn't produce enough insulin or becomes resistant to the effects of insulin, leading to elevated blood sugar levels.

Causes

The exact cause of type 2 diabetes is not fully understood, but several factors contribute to its development:

1. **Genetics**: Family history plays a significant role in predisposing individuals to type 2 diabetes. Certain genetic variations can increase the risk of developing the condition.

2. **Obesity**: Excess body weight, particularly abdominal fat, is strongly associated with insulin resistance and type 2 diabetes. Adipose tissue, especially visceral fat, releases inflammatory substances that interfere with insulin action.

3. **Physical Inactivity**: Lack of regular physical activity can contribute to obesity and insulin resistance, increasing the risk of type 2 diabetes. Exercise helps improve insulin sensitivity and glucose utilization by muscle cells.

4. **Unhealthy Diet**: A diet high in refined carbohydrates, sugars, and saturated fats can contribute to insulin resistance and obesity, increasing the risk of type 2 diabetes. Processed foods, sugary beverages, and excessive consumption of red meat are particularly problematic.

5. **Age**: The risk of type 2 diabetes increases with age, particularly after 45 years. This is partly due to reduced physical activity and muscle mass, as well as changes in hormone levels that affect glucose metabolism.

6. **Ethnicity**: Certain ethnic groups, such as African Americans, Hispanics, Native Americans, and Asian Americans, have a higher risk of developing type 2 diabetes compared to Caucasians. Genetic predisposition and lifestyle factors contribute to these disparities.

Symptoms

Type 2 diabetes often develops gradually, and some individuals may not experience noticeable symptoms initially. Common symptoms include:

- **Increased thirst**: Excessive thirst (polydipsia) is often one of the earliest signs of diabetes as the body tries to flush out excess sugar through urine.

- **Frequent urination**: Excess glucose in the bloodstream leads to increased urine production, causing frequent urination (polyuria).

- **Fatigue**: Insufficient glucose uptake by cells results in reduced energy production, leading to fatigue and weakness.

- **Blurred vision**: High blood sugar levels can cause fluid imbalances in the eye, leading to blurred vision.

- **Slow wound healing**: Poorly controlled diabetes impairs the body's ability to heal wounds and infections.

- **Increased hunger**: Despite eating, individuals with diabetes may experience persistent hunger (polyphagia) due to cells' inability to utilize glucose effectively.

Risk Factors

Several factors increase the risk of developing type 2 diabetes:

- **Obesity**: Being overweight or obese significantly increases the risk of type 2 diabetes.

- **Family history**: Having a parent or sibling with type 2 diabetes increases the likelihood of developing the condition.

- **Physical inactivity**: Lack of regular exercise and sedentary lifestyle contribute to insulin resistance and diabetes risk.

- **Age**: The risk of type 2 diabetes increases with age, especially after 45 years.

- **Race and ethnicity**: Certain ethnic groups have a higher predisposition to type 2 diabetes.

- **Gestational diabetes**: Women who had gestational diabetes during pregnancy are at increased risk of developing type 2 diabetes later in life.

- **Polycystic ovary syndrome (PCOS)**: Women with PCOS are at higher risk of insulin resistance and type 2 diabetes.

- **Hypertension (high blood pressure)**: Having high blood pressure is associated with an increased risk of type 2 diabetes.

- **High cholesterol levels**: Elevated levels of LDL cholesterol and triglycerides are linked to insulin resistance and diabetes risk.

- **Smoking**: Tobacco use increases the risk of type 2 diabetes and complicates its management.

The Importance of Diet and Lifestyle in Managing Type 2 Diabetes

Diet and lifestyle modifications are fundamental pillars in the management of type 2 diabetes. These interventions aim to improve blood sugar control, reduce insulin resistance, promote weight loss, and lower the risk of diabetes-related complications. By adopting a healthy diet and active lifestyle, individuals with type 2 diabetes can enhance their overall health and well-being while reducing reliance on medications.

Dietary Strategies

1. **Carbohydrate Management**: Carbohydrates have the most significant impact on blood sugar levels, making carbohydrate management crucial for diabetes management. Focus on consuming complex carbohydrates with a low glycemic index (GI) to minimize blood sugar spikes. Examples include whole grains, legumes, vegetables, and fruits.

2. **Portion Control**: Controlling portion sizes helps regulate calorie intake and prevent blood sugar fluctuations. Use smaller plates and avoid oversized portions, especially of high-calorie foods.

3. **Balanced Meals**: Aim for balanced meals that include a combination of carbohydrates, protein, and healthy fats. This

helps slow down the absorption of carbohydrates, preventing rapid spikes in blood sugar levels.

4. **Fiber-Rich Foods**: Incorporate plenty of fiber-rich foods into your diet, such as vegetables, fruits, whole grains, and legumes. Fiber helps regulate blood sugar levels, improve satiety, and support digestive health.

5. **Healthy Fats**: Choose sources of unsaturated fats, such as avocados, nuts, seeds, and olive oil, over saturated and trans fats. Healthy fats help reduce inflammation, improve cholesterol levels, and support heart health.

6. **Limit Sugary Foods and Beverages**: Minimize consumption of sugary snacks, desserts, sodas, and sweetened beverages, as they can cause rapid spikes in blood sugar levels.

7. **Regular Meal Timing**: Consistency in meal timing helps stabilize blood sugar levels and optimize insulin sensitivity. Aim to eat meals and snacks at regular intervals throughout the day.

8. **Hydration**: Stay hydrated by drinking plenty of water throughout the day. Opt for water or unsweetened beverages over sugary drinks.

Physical Activity

Regular physical activity is essential for managing type 2 diabetes and improving overall health. Exercise helps lower blood sugar levels, improve insulin sensitivity, control weight, reduce cardiovascular risk factors, and enhance mood and well-being. Aim for at least 150 minutes of moderate-intensity aerobic activity, such as brisk walking, cycling, or swimming, per week, along with muscle-strengthening activities on two or more days per week. Incorporate activities you enjoy and find ways to stay active throughout the day, such as taking the stairs, gardening, or dancing.

Stress Management and Sleep

Chronic stress and inadequate sleep can negatively impact blood sugar control and overall health. Practice stress-reducing techniques such as deep breathing, meditation, yoga, or spending time in nature. Aim for 7-9 hours of quality sleep per night to support optimal health and well-being.

Monitoring and Medication

Regular monitoring of blood sugar levels is essential for assessing treatment effectiveness and making adjustments as needed. Your healthcare provider may prescribe medications to help lower blood sugar levels, improve insulin sensitivity, or manage other diabetes-related conditions such as high blood pressure or high cholesterol. It's essential to follow your treatment plan as prescribed and communicate any concerns or changes in symptoms to your healthcare team.

Key Principles of a Diabetes-Friendly Diet for Beginners

Adopting a diabetes-friendly diet can seem daunting at first, but with the right knowledge and guidance, it can become a sustainable and enjoyable way of eating. Here are some key principles to help beginners navigate the world of diabetes nutrition:

1. Focus on Whole, Unprocessed Foods

Base your meals around whole, unprocessed foods such as fruits, vegetables, whole grains, lean proteins, and healthy fats. These foods are rich in essential nutrients, fiber, and antioxidants, promoting overall health and blood sugar control.

2. Monitor Carbohydrate Intake

Carbohydrates have the most significant impact on blood sugar levels, so it's crucial to monitor your carbohydrate intake and choose wisely. Focus on complex carbohydrates with a low glycemic index (GI) to minimize blood sugar spikes. Examples include whole grains like quinoa, brown rice, oats, and legumes like lentils, chickpeas, and black beans.

3. Practice Portion Control

Controlling portion sizes helps regulate calorie intake and prevent overeating, which can lead to blood sugar fluctuations and weight gain. Use measuring cups, spoons, or visual cues to gauge appropriate portion sizes, and avoid oversized servings, especially of high-calorie foods.

4. Include Lean Proteins

Protein-rich foods help promote satiety, stabilize blood sugar levels, and support muscle health. Include lean sources of protein such as skinless poultry, fish, tofu, tempeh, legumes, and low-fat dairy products in your meals and snacks.

5. Choose Healthy Fats

Incorporate sources of healthy fats into your diet, such as avocados, nuts, seeds, olive oil, and fatty fish like salmon and mackerel. Healthy fats help reduce inflammation, improve cholesterol levels, and support heart health. Limit saturated and trans fats found in fried foods, processed snacks, and fatty meats.

6. Be Mindful of Sugars and Sweeteners

Limit added sugars and sweetened foods and beverages, as they can cause rapid spikes in blood sugar levels. Choose natural sweeteners like stevia, erythritol, or monk fruit in moderation, and opt for sugar-free or unsweetened alternatives whenever possible.

7. Stay Hydrated

Drink plenty of water throughout the day to stay hydrated and support optimal health. Limit sugary beverages like sodas, fruit juices, and sweetened teas, as they can contribute to excess calorie intake and blood sugar spikes.

8. Plan and Prepare Ahead

Meal planning and preparation can help you stay on track with your diabetes-friendly diet and avoid unhealthy food choices. Plan your meals and snacks in advance, make a grocery list, and stock up on nutritious ingredients. Prepare healthy meals and snacks ahead of time to have convenient options available when hunger strikes.

9. Seek Support and Education

Managing type 2 diabetes can be challenging, but you don't have to do it alone. Seek support from healthcare professionals, diabetes educators, support groups, or online communities to learn more about diabetes management, share experiences, and stay motivated on your journey to better health.

10. Be Patient and Persistent

Making lifestyle changes takes time and effort, so be patient with yourself and celebrate small victories along the way. Focus on progress rather than perfection, and remember that every positive choice you make contributes to your overall health and well-being. With consistency and perseverance, you can successfully manage type 2 diabetes and live a fulfilling life.

CHAPTER TWO

Getting Started with Type 2 Diabetes Cooking

Introduction to Diabetes-Friendly Ingredients and Substitutions

Cooking delicious and nutritious meals while managing type 2 diabetes is not only possible but also essential for maintaining optimal health. By understanding diabetes-friendly ingredients and making smart substitutions, you can create flavorful dishes that support blood sugar control and overall well-being.

1. Whole Grains

Whole grains are rich in fiber, vitamins, minerals, and complex carbohydrates, making them an excellent choice for individuals with type 2 diabetes. They help stabilize blood sugar levels, promote satiety, and support digestive health. Examples of whole grains include:

- Brown rice
- Quinoa
- Oats
- Barley
- Whole wheat
- Bulgur

- Farro

2. Lean Proteins

Incorporating lean proteins into your meals helps promote fullness, stabilize blood sugar levels, and support muscle health. Choose lean cuts of meat, poultry without skin, fish, seafood, tofu, tempeh, legumes, and low-fat dairy products. Opt for cooking methods such as grilling, baking, broiling, or steaming to minimize added fats.

3. Non-Starchy Vegetables

Non-starchy vegetables are low in calories and carbohydrates while high in fiber, vitamins, minerals, and antioxidants. They have a minimal impact on blood sugar levels and can be enjoyed in abundance. Include a variety of colorful vegetables in your meals, such as:

- Leafy greens (spinach, kale, arugula)
- Cruciferous vegetables (broccoli, cauliflower, Brussels sprouts)
- Bell peppers
- Tomatoes
- Cucumbers
- Zucchini

- Mushrooms
- Asparagus

4. Healthy Fats

Incorporating sources of healthy fats into your diet helps improve cholesterol levels, reduce inflammation, and support heart health. Choose unsaturated fats from plant-based sources such as:

- Avocado
- Nuts (almonds, walnuts, pistachios)
- Seeds (chia seeds, flaxseeds, pumpkin seeds)
- Olive oil
- Canola oil
- Fatty fish (salmon, mackerel, sardines)

Limit saturated and trans fats found in processed foods, fried foods, fatty meats, and full-fat dairy products.

5. Low-Glycemic Sweeteners

When sweetening foods and beverages, opt for low-glycemic sweeteners that have a minimal impact on blood sugar levels. Examples include:

- Stevia

- Erythritol
- Monk fruit
- Xylitol

Use these sweeteners in moderation and be mindful of portion sizes to avoid overconsumption.

6. Herbs and Spices

Herbs and spices are excellent flavor enhancers that can elevate the taste of your dishes without adding extra calories or sodium. Experiment with a variety of herbs and spices to add depth and complexity to your meals. Some diabetes-friendly options include:

- Cinnamon
- Turmeric
- Ginger
- Garlic
- Rosemary
- Thyme
- Basil
- Cumin
- Paprika

- Chili powder

Essential Kitchen Tools and Equipment for Beginner Cooks

Equipping your kitchen with essential tools and equipment can make cooking easier, more efficient, and enjoyable, especially if you're new to cooking or managing type 2 diabetes. Here are some must-have items for beginner cooks:

1. Chef's Knife

A sharp chef's knife is essential for chopping, slicing, dicing, and mincing ingredients with precision and ease. Invest in a high-quality chef's knife that feels comfortable and well-balanced in your hand.

2. Cutting Board

A durable cutting board provides a stable surface for chopping and preparing ingredients. Choose a cutting board made of wood, plastic, or bamboo that is large enough to accommodate your cooking needs and easy to clean.

3. Non-Stick Cookware

Non-stick pots and pans are ideal for cooking with minimal oil or fat, making them suitable for individuals with type 2 diabetes who are watching their fat intake. Look for non-stick cookware with a durable coating that is free of harmful chemicals such as PFOA and PTFE.

4. Baking Sheet

A baking sheet or sheet pan is versatile and can be used for roasting vegetables, baking proteins, or making sheet pan meals. Choose a sturdy baking sheet with raised edges to prevent spills and facilitate easy handling.

5. Measuring Cups and Spoons

Accurate measurement is crucial for achieving consistent results in cooking and baking. Invest in a set of measuring cups and spoons for precise portioning of ingredients.

6. Blender or Food Processor

A blender or food processor is handy for making smoothies, sauces, soups, dips, and dressings. Choose a blender with variable speed settings and a powerful motor for smooth and efficient blending.

7. Oven Thermometer

An oven thermometer ensures that your oven maintains the correct temperature for baking and roasting. This helps prevent undercooked or overcooked dishes and ensures even cooking.

8. Kitchen Scale

A kitchen scale is useful for measuring ingredients by weight, especially for baking recipes that require precise measurements. It allows for greater accuracy and consistency in cooking and baking.

9. Instant-Read Thermometer

An instant-read thermometer is essential for checking the internal temperature of cooked meats, poultry, and fish to ensure they are safely cooked and free from harmful bacteria.

Tips for Grocery Shopping and Meal Planning for Diabetes Management

Effective grocery shopping and meal planning are key components of successful diabetes management. By making thoughtful choices at the grocery store and planning ahead, you can create nutritious and satisfying meals that support blood sugar control and overall health.

1. Make a Shopping List

Before heading to the grocery store, make a list of the items you need based on your planned meals and recipes. Organize your list by categories such as produce, proteins, dairy, grains, and pantry staples to streamline your shopping trip.

2. Stick to the Perimeter

Focus on shopping for fresh, whole foods located around the perimeter of the grocery store, such as fruits, vegetables, lean proteins, dairy, and whole grains. Minimize purchases of processed and packaged foods found in the center aisles, which tend to be higher in added sugars, unhealthy fats, and sodium.

3. Read Food Labels

When choosing packaged foods, read food labels carefully to understand their nutritional content, including calories, carbohydrates, sugars, fiber, fats, and sodium. Look for products with minimal added sugars, saturated fats, and sodium, and prioritize items with high fiber content and whole food ingredients.

4. Choose Low-Glycemic Options

Select foods with a low glycemic index (GI), which have a slower impact on blood sugar levels and help maintain stable energy levels throughout the day. Examples of low-GI foods include non-starchy vegetables, legumes, whole grains, and lean proteins.

5. Plan Meals in Advance

Set aside time each week to plan your meals and snacks for the upcoming days. Consider your schedule, preferences, and nutritional needs when selecting recipes and creating your meal plan. Aim for a balance of carbohydrates, proteins, and healthy fats in each meal to support blood sugar control and satiety.

6. Batch Cook and Prep Ingredients

Spend time batch cooking and prepping ingredients in advance to save time and effort during the week. Cook grains, proteins, and vegetables in large batches and portion them into individual containers for easy reheating and assembly. Wash, chop, and store fruits and vegetables for quick and convenient snacks and meals.

7. Incorporate Variety and Flexibility

Keep your meals interesting and enjoyable by incorporating a variety of flavors, textures, and cuisines into your meal plan. Be flexible and open to trying new recipes, ingredients, and cooking techniques to keep your taste buds satisfied and motivated.

8. Stock Up on Staples

Keep your pantry, refrigerator, and freezer stocked with staple ingredients that can be used to create quick and easy meals on busy days. Some essential pantry staples for diabetes-friendly cooking include:

- Whole grains (brown rice, quinoa, oats)
- Canned beans and legumes
- Canned tomatoes and tomato sauce
- Olive oil and cooking oils

- Vinegar (balsamic, apple cider)
- Herbs and spices
- Nuts and seeds
- Low-sodium broth or stock

9. Practice Portion Control

Be mindful of portion sizes when serving meals and snacks to help regulate calorie intake and blood sugar levels. Use measuring cups, spoons, or visual cues to gauge appropriate portion sizes, and avoid oversized servings, especially of high-calorie foods.

10. Stay Organized and Consistent

Establish a routine for grocery shopping, meal planning, and meal preparation to stay organized and consistent with your diabetes management efforts. Set aside time each week to review your meal plan, make adjustments as needed, and ensure you have everything you need for successful cooking and eating. By prioritizing your health and well-being and making conscious choices in the kitchen, you can effectively manage type 2 diabetes and enjoy delicious meals that nourish your body and soul.

CHAPTER THREE

Breakfasts to Start Your Day Right

Quick and Healthy Breakfast Ideas for Busy Mornings

Mornings can be hectic, but starting your day with a nutritious breakfast sets the tone for better energy levels and productivity. Here are some quick and healthy breakfast ideas that are perfect for busy mornings:

1. Overnight Oats

Prepare a batch of overnight oats the night before by combining rolled oats with your choice of milk (dairy or plant-based), Greek yogurt, chia seeds, and a dash of sweetener (such as honey or maple syrup). Add flavorings like vanilla extract, cinnamon, or cocoa powder, and let it sit in the refrigerator overnight. In the morning, top with fresh fruit, nuts, or seeds for added texture and flavor.

2. Greek Yogurt Parfait

Layer Greek yogurt with fresh berries, sliced bananas, and a sprinkle of granola or chopped nuts in a glass or bowl to create a delicious parfait. Greek yogurt is rich in protein, calcium, and probiotics, while fruits and nuts add fiber, vitamins, and healthy fats.

3. Whole Grain Toast with Nut Butter

Toast a slice of whole grain bread and spread it with your favorite nut butter (such as almond, peanut, or cashew butter). Top with sliced fruit (such as bananas or strawberries) or a drizzle of honey for extra sweetness. Whole grain bread provides complex carbohydrates and fiber, while nut butter adds protein and healthy fats to keep you satisfied until your next meal.

4. Smoothie Bowl

Blend together frozen fruits (such as berries, mango, or pineapple), leafy greens (such as spinach or kale), Greek yogurt or protein powder, and a liquid base (such as almond milk or coconut water) until smooth. Pour the smoothie into a bowl and top with toppings like granola, sliced fruit, nuts, seeds, or shredded coconut for added nutrition and texture.

5. Veggie Omelette or Scramble

Whisk together eggs or egg whites with diced vegetables (such as bell peppers, onions, spinach, tomatoes, or mushrooms) and a sprinkle of cheese (optional). Cook the mixture in a non-stick skillet until set, then fold it over to create an omelette or scramble. Serve with whole grain toast or a side of fruit for a balanced meal.

6. Cottage Cheese with Fruit

Top a serving of cottage cheese with sliced fruit (such as pineapple, peaches, or berries) and a sprinkle of nuts or seeds for added crunch. Cottage cheese is high in protein and calcium, while fruit provides natural sweetness and fiber.

7. Breakfast Wrap or Burrito

Fill a whole grain tortilla with scrambled eggs, black beans, diced avocado, salsa, and shredded cheese for a satisfying breakfast wrap or burrito. Roll it up tightly and enjoy it on the go or as a sit-down meal with a side of fresh fruit.

8. Chia Seed Pudding

Mix chia seeds with your choice of milk (such as almond milk or coconut milk) and a touch of sweetener (such as honey or agave syrup) in a jar or bowl. Let it sit in the refrigerator for at least 30 minutes or overnight until it thickens into a pudding-like consistency. Top with fresh fruit, nuts, or coconut flakes before serving.

9. Breakfast Muffins or Bars

Bake a batch of homemade breakfast muffins or bars packed with oats, nuts, seeds, dried fruit, and spices for a convenient grab-and-go option. Make them ahead of time and store them in an airtight container for a quick and portable breakfast or snack.

10. Protein-Packed Smoothie

Blend together protein-rich ingredients such as Greek yogurt, protein powder, spinach, avocado, and almond butter with frozen fruits and a liquid base (such as almond milk or coconut water) for a filling and nutritious smoothie. Customize the flavor and texture by adding your favorite mix-ins like cocoa powder, vanilla extract, or spices.

These quick and healthy breakfast ideas are perfect for busy mornings when you need a nutritious and satisfying meal to fuel your day. With a little planning and creativity, you can enjoy a delicious breakfast that supports your health and well-being, even on the busiest of days.

High-Fiber Breakfasts to Regulate Blood Sugar Levels

Starting your day with a high-fiber breakfast can help regulate blood sugar levels, improve digestion, and promote satiety. Fiber-rich foods slow down the absorption of sugar into the bloodstream, preventing rapid spikes and crashes in blood glucose levels. Here are some high-fiber breakfast ideas to try:

1. Oatmeal with Fruit and Nuts

Prepare a bowl of oatmeal using rolled oats and your choice of milk (dairy or plant-based). Top it with sliced fruit (such as berries, bananas, or apples) and a sprinkle of nuts or seeds (such as almonds, walnuts, or chia seeds) for added fiber, vitamins, and healthy fats.

2. Whole Grain Toast with Avocado and Eggs

Toast a slice of whole grain bread and top it with mashed avocado and a cooked egg (such as scrambled, poached, or fried). Avocado is rich in fiber, healthy fats, and vitamins, while eggs provide protein and essential nutrients.

3. Chia Seed Pudding with Berries

Mix chia seeds with your choice of milk (such as almond milk or coconut milk) and a touch of sweetener (such as honey or maple syrup) in a jar or bowl. Let it sit in the refrigerator until it thickens into a pudding-like consistency. Top with fresh berries for added flavor, fiber, and antioxidants.

4. Greek Yogurt with Granola and Fruit

Enjoy a serving of Greek yogurt with a sprinkle of granola (choose a low-sugar, high-fiber variety) and fresh fruit (such as kiwi, pineapple, or pomegranate seeds) for a creamy and satisfying breakfast packed with protein, fiber, and nutrients.

5. Smoothie with Leafy Greens and Flaxseeds

Blend together leafy greens (such as spinach or kale), frozen fruit (such as mango or pineapple), Greek yogurt or protein powder, flaxseeds or chia seeds, and a liquid base (such as water or coconut water) until smooth. Green smoothies are a convenient way to increase your fiber intake and boost your morning nutrition.

6. Whole Grain Pancakes or Waffles with Nut Butter

Make a batch of whole grain pancakes or waffles using whole wheat flour or oat flour. Top them with a dollop of nut butter (such as almond butter or peanut butter) and sliced fruit (such as bananas or strawberries) for a fiber-rich and delicious breakfast.

7. Veggie Breakfast Burrito or Wrap

Fill a whole grain tortilla with scrambled eggs, black beans, sautéed vegetables (such as bell peppers, onions, and spinach), and salsa for a hearty and fiber-packed breakfast burrito or wrap. Wrap it up tightly and enjoy it on the go or as a sit-down meal.

8. Quinoa Breakfast Bowl with Nuts and Seeds

Cook quinoa according to package instructions and serve it warm or cold in a bowl. Top it with chopped nuts (such as almonds or walnuts), seeds (such as pumpkin seeds or sunflower seeds), and dried fruit (such as raisins or apricots) for a protein-rich and fiber-filled breakfast option.

9. Bran Muffins or Bars

Bake homemade bran muffins or bars using whole grain flour, wheat bran, oats, nuts, seeds, and dried fruit. These fiber-rich breakfast treats are perfect for meal prep and can be enjoyed on busy mornings or as a portable snack throughout the day.

10. High-Fiber Cereal with Milk and Fruit

Choose a high-fiber cereal with at least 5 grams of fiber per serving and pair it with your choice of milk (such as dairy or plant-based) and fresh fruit (such as berries or sliced peaches) for a quick and easy breakfast that's rich in fiber and nutrients.

Incorporating high-fiber foods into your breakfast routine can help regulate blood sugar levels, support digestive health, and keep you feeling full and satisfied until your next meal. Experiment with different combinations and flavors to find your favorite high-fiber breakfast options.

Protein-Packed Breakfasts to Keep You Full and Energized

Starting your day with a protein-packed breakfast can help keep you full, satisfied, and energized until your next meal. Protein helps stabilize blood sugar levels, promotes muscle repair and growth, and supports overall health and well-being. Here are some protein-packed breakfast ideas to try:

1. Eggs with Whole Grain Toast and Avocado

Cook eggs (such as scrambled, poached, or fried) and serve them with whole grain toast and sliced avocado for a balanced and satisfying breakfast. Eggs are rich in high-quality protein, vitamins, and minerals, while avocado provides healthy fats and fiber.

2. Greek Yogurt with Nuts and Berries

Enjoy a serving of Greek yogurt topped with chopped nuts (such as almonds, walnuts, or pecans) and fresh berries (such as strawberries, blueberries, or raspberries) for a creamy and protein-rich breakfast. Greek yogurt is higher in protein and lower in sugar compared to regular yogurt, making it an excellent choice for breakfast.

3. Protein Smoothie with Spinach and Nut Butter

Blend together protein powder, leafy greens (such as spinach or kale), frozen fruit (such as bananas or berries), nut butter (such as almond butter or peanut butter), and a liquid base (such as almond milk or coconut water) until smooth. Protein smoothies are a convenient way to increase your protein intake and boost your morning nutrition.

4. Cottage Cheese with Pineapple and Seeds

Serve cottage cheese with diced pineapple and a sprinkle of seeds (such as chia seeds, flaxseeds, or pumpkin seeds) for a protein-rich and refreshing breakfast option. Cottage cheese is high in protein and calcium, while pineapple provides natural sweetness and vitamin C.

5. Breakfast Burrito or Wrap with Beans and Cheese

Fill a whole grain tortilla with scrambled eggs, black beans, shredded cheese, and salsa for a hearty and protein-packed breakfast burrito or wrap. Beans are an excellent plant-based source of protein and fiber, while eggs and cheese provide additional protein and essential nutrients.

6. Protein Pancakes or Waffles with Fruit and Yogurt

Make a batch of protein pancakes or waffles using protein powder, whole wheat flour, oats, or almond flour. Top them with sliced fruit (such as bananas or berries) and a dollop of Greek yogurt for added protein and flavor. Drizzle with honey or maple syrup if desired.

7. Smoked Salmon and Cream Cheese Bagel

Spread cream cheese on a whole grain bagel and top it with smoked salmon, sliced tomatoes, red onion, and capers for a protein-rich and satisfying breakfast option. Smoked salmon is rich in omega-3 fatty acids, while cream cheese adds creaminess and flavor.

8. Tofu Scramble with Vegetables

Sauté tofu with diced vegetables (such as bell peppers, onions, spinach, and mushrooms) and seasonings (such as turmeric, garlic powder, and nutritional yeast) for a plant-based alternative to scrambled eggs. Tofu is a versatile source of protein that can be flavored and seasoned to your liking.

9. Protein-Packed Muffins or Bars

Bake homemade muffins or bars using protein powder, oats, nuts, seeds, and dried fruit for a convenient and portable breakfast option. These protein-packed treats are perfect for meal prep and can be enjoyed on busy mornings or as a post-workout snack.

10. High-Protein Cereal with Milk and Nut Butter

Choose a high-protein cereal with at least 10 grams of protein per serving and pair it with your choice of milk (such as dairy or plant-based) and a dollop of nut butter (such as almond butter or cashew butter) for added protein and flavor. Sprinkle with cinnamon or cocoa powder for extra sweetness.

Incorporating protein-rich foods into your breakfast routine can help keep you feeling full, satisfied, and energized throughout the day. Experiment with different combinations and flavors to find your favorite protein-packed breakfast options that suit your taste preferences and dietary needs.

CHAPTER FOUR

Simple and Satisfying Lunches

Easy Salad and Wrap Recipes for Balanced Lunches

Salads and wraps offer a delightful mix of flavors, textures, and nutrients, making them perfect for a satisfying and balanced lunch. Here are some effortless recipes to try:

Mediterranean Quinoa Salad:

Ingredients:

- 1 cup quinoa, cooked
- 1 cucumber, diced
- 1 cup cherry tomatoes, halved
- 1/4 cup Kalamata olives, sliced
- 1/4 cup red onion, finely chopped
- 1/4 cup crumbled feta cheese
- 2 tablespoons fresh lemon juice
- 2 tablespoons extra virgin olive oil
- 2 tablespoons chopped fresh parsley
- Salt and pepper to taste

Instructions:

1. In a large bowl, combine cooked quinoa, diced cucumber, halved cherry tomatoes, sliced Kalamata olives, chopped red onion, and crumbled feta cheese.

2. Drizzle with fresh lemon juice and extra virgin olive oil.

3. Add chopped fresh parsley and season with salt and pepper to taste.

4. Toss gently to combine all ingredients.

5. Serve chilled or at room temperature as a refreshing and nutritious salad.

Turkey and Avocado Wrap:

Ingredients:

- 1 large whole grain tortilla
- 3 slices deli turkey breast
- 1/4 avocado, sliced
- 1/4 cup mixed greens
- 1 tablespoon hummus
- 1 teaspoon Dijon mustard

Instructions:

1. Lay the whole grain tortilla flat on a clean surface.

2. Spread hummus and Dijon mustard evenly over the tortilla.

3. Layer slices of deli turkey breast, avocado slices, and mixed greens on top of the tortilla.

4. Roll up the tortilla tightly to form a wrap.

5. Slice the wrap in half diagonally and serve immediately or pack for lunch on the go.

Asian Chicken Salad:

Ingredients:

- 2 cups shredded rotisserie chicken
- 4 cups mixed salad greens
- 1/2 cup shredded carrots
- 1/2 cup sliced cucumber
- 1/4 cup sliced almonds
- 2 tablespoons chopped fresh cilantro
- 2 tablespoons sesame seeds
- 1/4 cup Asian ginger dressing

Instructions:

1. In a large bowl, combine shredded rotisserie chicken, mixed salad greens, shredded carrots, sliced cucumber, sliced almonds, chopped fresh cilantro, and sesame seeds.

2. Drizzle with Asian ginger dressing and toss gently to coat.

3. Serve immediately as a flavorful and satisfying salad option.

Caprese Wrap:

Ingredients:

- 1 large whole grain tortilla
- 1/2 cup fresh mozzarella balls, halved
- 1/2 cup cherry tomatoes, halved
- 1/4 cup fresh basil leaves
- 1 tablespoon balsamic glaze
- Salt and pepper to taste

Instructions:

1. Lay the whole grain tortilla flat on a clean surface.

2. Arrange fresh mozzarella balls, halved cherry tomatoes, and fresh basil leaves in the center of the tortilla.

3. Drizzle with balsamic glaze and season with salt and pepper to taste.

4. Roll up the tortilla tightly to form a wrap.

5. Slice the wrap in half diagonally and serve immediately or pack for lunch.

Flavorful Soup and Sandwich Combos for Comforting Meals

Soup and sandwich combos are classic comfort foods that offer a satisfying and flavorful meal. Here are some delightful combinations to enjoy:

Tomato Basil Soup with Grilled Cheese Sandwich:

Ingredients for Tomato Basil Soup:

- 2 tablespoons olive oil
- 1 onion, chopped
- 2 cloves garlic, minced
- 1 can (28 ounces) whole tomatoes, undrained
- 2 cups vegetable broth
- 1/2 cup fresh basil leaves, chopped
- Salt and pepper to taste
- 1/2 cup heavy cream (optional)

Instructions:

1. In a large pot, heat olive oil over medium heat.
2. Add chopped onion and minced garlic, and cook until softened.
3. Add whole tomatoes with their juices and vegetable broth to the pot.
4. Bring to a simmer and cook for about 15 minutes.
5. Stir in chopped basil leaves and season with salt and pepper to taste.
6. Use an immersion blender to puree the soup until smooth.
7. If desired, stir in heavy cream for added creaminess.
8. Serve hot with grilled cheese sandwiches on the side.

Ingredients for Grilled Cheese Sandwich:

- 4 slices whole grain bread
- 4 slices cheddar cheese
- Butter

Instructions:

1. Heat a skillet over medium heat.
2. Butter one side of each slice of bread.

3. Place a slice of cheddar cheese on the unbuttered side of two bread slices.

4. Top with the remaining bread slices, buttered side facing out.

5. Place sandwiches in the skillet and cook until golden brown on both sides and the cheese is melted.

6. Slice each sandwich in half and serve alongside tomato basil soup.

Chicken Noodle Soup with Turkey Club Sandwich:

Ingredients for Chicken Noodle Soup:

- 1 tablespoon olive oil
- 1 onion, chopped
- 2 carrots, sliced
- 2 celery stalks, sliced
- 2 cloves garlic, minced
- 6 cups chicken broth
- 2 cups shredded cooked chicken
- 2 cups egg noodles
- Salt and pepper to taste

- Fresh parsley, chopped (for garnish)

Instructions:

1. In a large pot, heat olive oil over medium heat.
2. Add chopped onion, sliced carrots, sliced celery, and minced garlic to the pot.
3. Cook until vegetables are softened, about 5 minutes.
4. Pour in chicken broth and bring to a boil.
5. Add shredded cooked chicken and egg noodles to the pot.
6. Simmer until noodles are tender, about 8-10 minutes.
7. Season with salt and pepper to taste.
8. Serve hot, garnished with chopped fresh parsley.

Ingredients for Turkey Club Sandwich:

- 6 slices whole grain bread
- 6 slices cooked turkey bacon
- 6 slices roasted turkey breast
- 6 lettuce leaves
- 6 tomato slices
- Mayonnaise
- Mustard

Instructions:

1. Toast the whole grain bread slices until lightly golden.
2. Spread mayonnaise and mustard on one side of each bread slice.
3. Layer cooked turkey bacon, roasted turkey breast, lettuce leaves, and tomato slices on three slices of bread.
4. Top with the remaining bread slices, mayo and mustard side facing down.
5. Cut each sandwich in half diagonally and serve alongside chicken noodle soup.

Creamy Butternut Squash Soup with Turkey and Cranberry Panini:

Ingredients for Creamy Butternut Squash Soup:

- 1 butternut squash, peeled, seeded, and diced
- 1 onion, chopped
- 2 cloves garlic, minced
- 4 cups vegetable broth
- 1/2 cup coconut milk
- 1 tablespoon olive oil
- Salt and pepper to taste

Instructions:

1. In a large pot, heat olive oil over medium heat.
2. Add chopped onion and minced garlic, and cook until softened.
3. Add diced butternut squash and vegetable broth to the pot.
4. Bring to a boil, then reduce heat and simmer until squash is tender, about 20 minutes.
5. Use an immersion blender to puree the soup until smooth.
6. Stir in coconut milk and season with salt and pepper to taste.
7. Serve hot.

Ingredients for Turkey and Cranberry Panini:

- 8 slices whole grain bread
- 8 slices roasted turkey breast
- 1/2 cup cranberry sauce
- 4 slices Swiss cheese
- Butter

Instructions:

1. Heat a panini press or skillet over medium heat.
2. Spread cranberry sauce on one side of each bread slice.

3. Layer roasted turkey breast and Swiss cheese on four slices of bread.

4. Top with the remaining bread slices, cranberry sauce side down.

5. Spread butter on the outside of each sandwich.

6. Place sandwiches in the panini press or skillet and cook until golden brown and the cheese is melted.

7. Cut each sandwich in half diagonally and serve with creamy butternut squash soup.

Budget-Friendly Lunch Ideas for Work or School

Eating delicious and nutritious lunches on a budget is achievable with some creativity and planning. Here are some wallet-friendly ideas:

Rice and Bean Burrito Bowl:

Ingredients:

- 1 cup cooked rice
- 1 cup canned black beans, rinsed and drained
- 1/2 cup salsa
- 1/2 avocado, sliced
- 1/4 cup shredded cheese

- Fresh cilantro, chopped
- Lime wedges
- Salt and pepper to taste

Instructions:

1. In a microwave-safe container, layer cooked rice, black beans, salsa, sliced avocado, and shredded cheese.
2. Season with salt and pepper to taste.
3. Cover and refrigerate until ready to eat.
4. Heat in the microwave at work or school and garnish with chopped fresh cilantro and lime wedges before serving.

Pasta Salad with Vegetables:

Ingredients:

- 2 cups cooked pasta
- 1 cup cherry tomatoes, halved
- 1/2 cucumber, diced
- 1/2 bell pepper, diced
- 1/4 red onion, thinly sliced
- 1/4 cup Italian dressing
- Salt and pepper to taste

Instructions:

1. In a large bowl, combine cooked pasta, cherry tomatoes, diced cucumber, diced bell pepper, and thinly sliced red onion.

2. Toss with Italian dressing until well coated.

3. Season with salt and pepper to taste.

4. Divide into individual containers and refrigerate until ready to eat.

Veggie Stir-Fry with Rice:

Ingredients:

- 1 cup cooked rice
- 1 cup mixed vegetables (fresh or frozen)
- 1/2 cup firm tofu, diced
- 2 tablespoons soy sauce
- 1 tablespoon olive oil
- 1 clove garlic, minced
- 1 teaspoon grated ginger
- Salt and pepper to taste

Instructions:

1. In a skillet, heat olive oil over medium heat.
2. Add minced garlic and grated ginger, and sauté until fragrant.
3. Add mixed vegetables and diced tofu to the skillet.
4. Stir-fry until vegetables are tender-crisp.
5. Season with soy sauce, salt, and pepper to taste.
6. Serve over cooked rice and pack in a container for lunch.

Chickpea Salad Sandwich:

Ingredients:

- 1 can (15 ounces) chickpeas, drained and rinsed
- 1/4 cup diced celery
- 2 tablespoons diced red onion
- 2 tablespoons mayonnaise
- 1 tablespoon Dijon mustard
- 1 tablespoon lemon juice
- Salt and pepper to taste
- 4 slices whole grain bread
- Lettuce leaves
- Tomato slices

Instructions:

1. In a bowl, mash chickpeas with a fork until slightly chunky.
2. Add diced celery, diced red onion, mayonnaise, Dijon mustard, lemon juice, salt, and pepper to the bowl.
3. Stir until well combined and adjust seasoning to taste.
4. Spread chickpea salad onto whole grain bread slices.
5. Top with lettuce leaves and tomato slices to make sandwiches.
6. Wrap sandwiches in parchment paper or plastic wrap and refrigerate until ready to eat.

Vegetable Frittata Muffins:

Ingredients:

- 6 large eggs
- 1/2 cup mixed vegetables (such as bell peppers, onions, spinach, mushrooms)
- 1/4 cup shredded cheese
- 2 tablespoons milk (optional)
- Salt and pepper to taste

Instructions:

1. Preheat the oven to 375°F (190°C). Grease a muffin tin.
2. In a bowl, whisk together eggs, mixed vegetables, shredded cheese, milk (if using), salt, and pepper.
3. Pour the egg mixture evenly into the muffin tin.
4. Bake for 20-25 minutes or until the frittata muffins are set and golden brown.
5. Let cool slightly before removing from the muffin tin.
6. Pack in a container for lunch.

CHAPTER FIVE

Flavorful Dinners in a Flash

One-Pot Dinners for Minimal Cleanup and Maximum Flavor

One-pot dinners are a lifesaver on busy evenings when you want a delicious meal without spending hours in the kitchen or dealing with a pile of dishes afterward. These recipes combine all the elements of a satisfying dinner into a single pot, minimizing cleanup while maximizing flavor. Here are some delightful one-pot dinner ideas:

Chicken and Vegetable Stir-Fry:

Ingredients:

- 1 tablespoon sesame oil
- 1 pound boneless, skinless chicken breasts, thinly sliced
- 2 cups mixed vegetables (such as bell peppers, broccoli, carrots)
- 3 cloves garlic, minced
- 1 tablespoon grated ginger
- 1/4 cup low-sodium soy sauce
- 2 tablespoons hoisin sauce

- 2 green onions, sliced
- Cooked rice or noodles, for serving

Instructions:

1. Heat sesame oil in a large skillet or wok over medium-high heat.
2. Add sliced chicken breasts and cook until browned and cooked through.
3. Add mixed vegetables, minced garlic, and grated ginger to the skillet. Stir-fry for 3-4 minutes until vegetables are tender-crisp.
4. In a small bowl, whisk together low-sodium soy sauce and hoisin sauce. Pour over the chicken and vegetables in the skillet.
5. Stir to coat evenly and cook for an additional 2-3 minutes.
6. Garnish with sliced green onions and serve hot over cooked rice or noodles.

Creamy Mushroom Risotto:

Ingredients:

- 2 tablespoons butter
- 1 onion, finely chopped

- 2 cloves garlic, minced
- 1 cup Arborio rice
- 4 cups vegetable or chicken broth, heated
- 1 cup sliced mushrooms
- 1/4 cup grated Parmesan cheese
- Salt and pepper to taste
- Chopped fresh parsley, for garnish

Instructions:

1. In a large pot, melt butter over medium heat.
2. Add finely chopped onion and minced garlic to the pot. Cook until softened, about 2-3 minutes.
3. Add Arborio rice to the pot and stir to coat in the butter mixture.
4. Gradually add heated broth to the pot, one ladleful at a time, stirring frequently and allowing the rice to absorb the liquid before adding more.
5. Continue adding broth and stirring until the rice is creamy and tender, about 20-25 minutes.
6. Stir in sliced mushrooms and cook for an additional 3-4 minutes until mushrooms are tender.

7. Remove from heat and stir in grated Parmesan cheese. Season with salt and pepper to taste.

8. Garnish with chopped fresh parsley before serving.

Beef and Vegetable Stew:

Ingredients:

- 1 tablespoon olive oil
- 1 pound stewing beef, cut into bite-sized pieces
- 1 onion, chopped
- 2 carrots, sliced
- 2 celery stalks, sliced
- 2 cloves garlic, minced
- 4 cups beef broth
- 1 can (14.5 ounces) diced tomatoes
- 2 potatoes, peeled and diced
- 1 cup frozen peas
- 1 teaspoon dried thyme
- Salt and pepper to taste

Instructions:

1. Heat olive oil in a large pot or Dutch oven over medium heat.

2. Add stewing beef to the pot and cook until browned on all sides.

3. Add chopped onion, sliced carrots, sliced celery, and minced garlic to the pot. Cook until vegetables are softened, about 5 minutes.

4. Pour beef broth and diced tomatoes (with their juices) into the pot. Stir to combine.

5. Add diced potatoes, frozen peas, and dried thyme to the pot. Season with salt and pepper to taste.

6. Bring the stew to a boil, then reduce heat and simmer for 1-2 hours until beef is tender and flavors are well combined.

7. Serve hot, garnished with chopped fresh parsley if desired.

Quick and Easy Stir-Fries for Busy Evenings

Stir-fries are perfect for busy evenings when you need a quick and nutritious meal on the table in no time. These recipes are versatile, allowing you to use whatever ingredients you have on hand. Here are some quick and easy stir-fry ideas:

Shrimp and Vegetable Stir-Fry:

Ingredients:

- 1 tablespoon vegetable oil
- 1 pound shrimp, peeled and deveined

- 2 cups mixed vegetables (such as bell peppers, snap peas, broccoli)
- 3 cloves garlic, minced
- 1 tablespoon grated ginger
- 1/4 cup low-sodium soy sauce
- 2 tablespoons oyster sauce
- Cooked rice or noodles, for serving

Instructions:

1. Heat vegetable oil in a large skillet or wok over medium-high heat.
2. Add shrimp to the skillet and cook until pink and opaque, about 2-3 minutes per side. Remove from skillet and set aside.
3. Add mixed vegetables, minced garlic, and grated ginger to the skillet. Stir-fry for 3-4 minutes until vegetables are tender-crisp.
4. Return cooked shrimp to the skillet.
5. In a small bowl, whisk together low-sodium soy sauce and oyster sauce. Pour over the shrimp and vegetables in the skillet.
6. Stir to coat evenly and cook for an additional 2-3 minutes.

7. Serve hot over cooked rice or noodles.

Beef and Broccoli Stir-Fry:

Ingredients:

- 1 tablespoon sesame oil
- 1 pound flank steak, thinly sliced
- 2 cups broccoli florets
- 1 red bell pepper, sliced
- 3 cloves garlic, minced
- 1/4 cup low-sodium soy sauce
- 2 tablespoons hoisin sauce
- 2 green onions, sliced
- Cooked rice or noodles, for serving

Instructions:

1. Heat sesame oil in a large skillet or wok over medium-high heat.
2. Add thinly sliced flank steak to the skillet and cook until browned, about 2-3 minutes per side. Remove from skillet and set aside.

3. Add broccoli florets, sliced red bell pepper, and minced garlic to the skillet. Stir-fry for 3-4 minutes until vegetables are tender-crisp.

4. Return cooked flank steak to the skillet.

5. In a small bowl, whisk together low-sodium soy sauce and hoisin sauce. Pour over the beef and vegetables in the skillet.

6. Stir to coat evenly and cook for an additional 2-3 minutes.

7. Serve hot over cooked rice or noodles.

Vegetable Tofu Stir-Fry:

Ingredients:

- 1 tablespoon vegetable oil
- 1 block firm tofu, diced
- 2 cups mixed vegetables (such as bell peppers, snow peas, carrots)
- 3 cloves garlic, minced
- 1 tablespoon grated ginger
- 1/4 cup low-sodium soy sauce
- 1 tablespoon rice vinegar
- 1 tablespoon honey

- Cooked rice or noodles, for serving

Instructions:

1. Heat vegetable oil in a large skillet or wok over medium-high heat.

2. Add diced tofu to the skillet and cook until golden brown on all sides. Remove from skillet and set aside.

3. Add mixed vegetables, minced garlic, and grated ginger to the skillet. Stir-fry for 3-4 minutes until vegetables are tender-crisp.

4. Return cooked tofu to the skillet.

5. In a small bowl, whisk together low-sodium soy sauce, rice vinegar, and honey. Pour over the tofu and vegetables in the skillet.

6. Stir to coat evenly and cook for an additional 2-3 minutes.

7. Serve hot over cooked rice or noodles.

Comforting Casseroles and Skillet Meals for Weeknight Dinners

Casseroles and skillet meals are comforting and convenient options for weeknight dinners. They're easy to prepare and can be customized with your favorite ingredients. Here are some comforting casserole and skillet meal ideas:

Chicken and Rice Casserole:

Ingredients:

- 1 tablespoon olive oil
- 1 onion, chopped
- 2 cloves garlic, minced
- 1 pound boneless, skinless chicken breasts, diced
- 1 cup long-grain white rice
- 2 cups chicken broth
- 1 cup frozen mixed vegetables
- 1/2 cup shredded cheddar cheese
- Salt and pepper to taste

Instructions:

1. Preheat the oven to 375°F (190°C). Grease a 9x13-inch baking dish.
2. Heat olive oil in a skillet over medium heat.
3. Add chopped onion and minced garlic to the skillet. Cook until softened, about 2-3 minutes.
4. Add diced chicken breasts to the skillet and cook until browned on all sides.

5. Stir in long-grain white rice and chicken broth. Bring to a simmer.

6. Transfer the chicken and rice mixture to the prepared baking dish.

7. Sprinkle frozen mixed vegetables and shredded cheddar cheese over the top.

8. Cover the baking dish with foil and bake in the preheated oven for 30-35 minutes or until rice is cooked through and chicken is tender.

9. Remove foil and broil for an additional 2-3 minutes until cheese is bubbly and golden brown.

10. Serve hot.

Beef and Potato Skillet:

Ingredients:

- 1 tablespoon olive oil
- 1 onion, chopped
- 1 pound ground beef
- 3 russet potatoes, peeled and diced
- 1 cup beef broth
- 1 teaspoon paprika

- 1/2 teaspoon dried thyme
- Salt and pepper to taste
- Chopped fresh parsley, for garnish

Instructions:

1. Heat olive oil in a large skillet over medium heat.
2. Add chopped onion to the skillet and cook until softened, about 2-3 minutes.
3. Add ground beef to the skillet and cook until browned, breaking it up with a spoon.
4. Stir in diced russet potatoes, beef broth, paprika, dried thyme, salt, and pepper.
5. Cover and simmer for 15-20 minutes until potatoes are tender, stirring occasionally.
6. Remove from heat and garnish with chopped fresh parsley before serving.

Vegetarian Enchilada Casserole:

Ingredients:

- 1 tablespoon olive oil
- 1 onion, chopped
- 2 cloves garlic, minced

- 1 bell pepper, diced
- 1 zucchini, diced
- 1 can (15 ounces) black beans, drained and rinsed
- 1 can (15 ounces) corn kernels, drained
- 1 can (15 ounces) enchilada sauce
- 6 large flour tortillas
- 2 cups shredded Mexican cheese blend
- Chopped fresh cilantro, for garnish

Instructions:

1. Preheat the oven to 375°F (190°C). Grease a 9x13-inch baking dish.
2. Heat olive oil in a skillet over medium heat.
3. Add chopped onion and minced garlic to the skillet. Cook until softened, about 2-3 minutes.
4. Add diced bell pepper and diced zucchini to the skillet. Cook for an additional 3-4 minutes until vegetables are tender.
5. Stir in black beans, corn kernels, and enchilada sauce. Cook for 2-3 minutes until heated through.
6. Spread a thin layer of the vegetable mixture in the bottom of the prepared baking dish.

7. Place flour tortillas on top of the vegetable mixture, overlapping as needed.

8. Spoon remaining vegetable mixture over the tortillas.

9. Sprinkle shredded Mexican cheese blend over the top.

10. Cover the baking dish with foil and bake in the preheated oven for 20-25 minutes or until cheese is melted and bubbly.

11. Remove foil and broil for an additional 2-3 minutes until cheese is golden brown.

12. Garnish with chopped fresh cilantro before serving.

CHAPTER SEVEN

Delicious Diabetic-Friendly Desserts

Lower-Sugar Dessert Recipes for Satisfying Sweet Cravings

Enjoying desserts while managing diabetes is possible with these lower-sugar recipes that are still incredibly satisfying:

Chocolate Avocado Mousse:

Ingredients:

- 2 ripe avocados
- 1/4 cup unsweetened cocoa powder
- 1/4 cup milk (almond milk or any other milk of your choice)
- 1 teaspoon vanilla extract
- 2-3 tablespoons honey or maple syrup (adjust to taste)
- Fresh berries, for garnish

Instructions:

1. Scoop the flesh of the ripe avocados into a blender or food processor.
2. Add unsweetened cocoa powder, milk, vanilla extract, and honey or maple syrup to the blender.

3. Blend until smooth and creamy, scraping down the sides of the blender as needed.

4. Taste and adjust sweetness if necessary by adding more honey or maple syrup.

5. Divide the mousse into serving cups and refrigerate for at least 1 hour to chill.

6. Serve topped with fresh berries for a delightful and guilt-free dessert.

Greek Yogurt Panna Cotta:

Ingredients:

- 2 cups plain Greek yogurt
- 1/4 cup milk (almond milk or any other milk of your choice)
- 2-3 tablespoons honey or maple syrup (adjust to taste)
- 1 teaspoon vanilla extract
- 2 teaspoons unflavored gelatin powder
- Fresh fruit compote or sliced fruit, for serving

Instructions:

1. In a small bowl, sprinkle gelatin powder over milk and let it sit for 5 minutes to bloom.

2. In a saucepan, heat Greek yogurt, honey or maple syrup, and vanilla extract over low heat, stirring continuously until smooth and slightly warm.

3. Remove from heat and whisk in the bloomed gelatin mixture until fully dissolved.

4. Divide the mixture among serving glasses or ramekins.

5. Refrigerate for at least 4 hours or until set.

6. Serve chilled with fresh fruit compote or sliced fruit on top.

Almond Flour Banana Bread:

Ingredients:

- 2 ripe bananas, mashed
- 2 eggs
- 1/4 cup coconut oil, melted
- 1/4 cup honey or maple syrup
- 1 teaspoon vanilla extract
- 2 cups almond flour
- 1 teaspoon baking powder
- 1/2 teaspoon baking soda
- 1/2 teaspoon ground cinnamon

- 1/4 teaspoon salt
- Chopped nuts or dark chocolate chips (optional)

Instructions:

1. Preheat the oven to 350°F (175°C). Grease a loaf pan with coconut oil or line with parchment paper.
2. In a large bowl, whisk together mashed bananas, eggs, melted coconut oil, honey or maple syrup, and vanilla extract until well combined.
3. In a separate bowl, combine almond flour, baking powder, baking soda, ground cinnamon, and salt.
4. Gradually add the dry ingredients to the wet ingredients, stirring until just combined.
5. Fold in chopped nuts or dark chocolate chips, if using.
6. Pour the batter into the prepared loaf pan and smooth the top with a spatula.
7. Bake for 40-45 minutes or until a toothpick inserted into the center comes out clean.
8. Allow the banana bread to cool in the pan for 10 minutes before transferring it to a wire rack to cool completely.
9. Slice and serve as a delicious and lower-sugar dessert option.

Fruit-Based Desserts That Are Naturally Sweet and Nutritious

Fruit-based desserts are naturally sweet and nutritious, making them perfect for satisfying sweet cravings without spiking blood sugar levels:

Berry Chia Seed Pudding:

Ingredients:

- 1/4 cup chia seeds
- 1 cup unsweetened almond milk (or any other milk of your choice)
- 1 tablespoon honey or maple syrup
- 1/2 teaspoon vanilla extract
- 1 cup mixed berries (such as strawberries, blueberries, raspberries)
- Fresh mint leaves, for garnish

Instructions:

1. In a bowl, whisk together chia seeds, almond milk, honey or maple syrup, and vanilla extract until well combined.
2. Cover and refrigerate for at least 2 hours or overnight, stirring occasionally, until the mixture thickens into a pudding-like consistency.

3. Once the chia seed pudding is ready, spoon it into serving glasses or bowls.

4. Top with mixed berries and garnish with fresh mint leaves.

5. Serve chilled as a refreshing and nutritious dessert option.

Grilled Pineapple with Coconut Yogurt:

Ingredients:

- 1 pineapple, peeled, cored, and sliced into rings
- 1 tablespoon coconut oil, melted
- 1 cup plain Greek yogurt or coconut yogurt
- 1 tablespoon honey or maple syrup
- Shredded coconut, for garnish

Instructions:

1. Preheat a grill or grill pan over medium-high heat.

2. Brush pineapple slices with melted coconut oil on both sides.

3. Grill pineapple slices for 2-3 minutes on each side until grill marks appear and pineapple is slightly caramelized.

4. In a small bowl, mix together Greek yogurt or coconut yogurt with honey or maple syrup.

5. Serve grilled pineapple slices with a dollop of coconut yogurt on top.

6. Garnish with shredded coconut before serving.

Baked Apples with Cinnamon and Walnuts:

Ingredients:

- 4 apples (such as Honeycrisp or Granny Smith), cored
- 2 tablespoons melted coconut oil or butter
- 2 tablespoons honey or maple syrup
- 1 teaspoon ground cinnamon
- 1/4 cup chopped walnuts

Instructions:

1. Preheat the oven to 375°F (190°C). Grease a baking dish with coconut oil or butter.

2. Place cored apples in the baking dish.

3. In a small bowl, mix together melted coconut oil or butter, honey or maple syrup, and ground cinnamon.

4. Drizzle the mixture over the apples, ensuring they are evenly coated.

5. Sprinkle chopped walnuts over the top.

6. Bake for 25-30 minutes or until apples are tender.

7. Serve baked apples warm, optionally topped with a scoop of Greek yogurt or a sprinkle of additional cinnamon.

Indulgent Treats Made Healthier with Smart Ingredient Swaps

Indulge in these treats made healthier with smart ingredient swaps, perfect for satisfying cravings without compromising on taste:

Oatmeal Chocolate Chip Cookies:

Ingredients:

- 1 cup old-fashioned oats
- 1 cup almond flour
- 1/2 teaspoon baking soda
- 1/4 teaspoon salt
- 1/4 cup coconut oil, melted
- 1/4 cup honey or maple syrup
- 1 egg
- 1 teaspoon vanilla extract
- 1/2 cup dark chocolate chips

Instructions:

1. Preheat the oven to 350°F (175°C). Line a baking sheet with parchment paper.

2. In a large bowl, combine old-fashioned oats, almond flour, baking soda, and salt.

3. In a separate bowl, whisk together melted coconut oil, honey or maple syrup, egg, and vanilla extract until well combined.

4. Add the wet ingredients to the dry ingredients and mix until a dough forms.

5. Fold in dark chocolate chips.

6. Drop rounded tablespoons of dough onto the prepared baking sheet, spacing them apart.

7. Flatten each cookie slightly with the back of a spoon.

8. Bake for 10-12 minutes or until golden brown.

9. Allow the cookies to cool on the baking sheet for 5 minutes before transferring them to a wire rack to cool completely.

Chia Seed Chocolate Pudding:

Ingredients:

- 1/4 cup chia seeds

- 1 cup unsweetened almond milk (or any other milk of your choice)
- 2 tablespoons unsweetened cocoa powder
- 2 tablespoons honey or maple syrup
- 1/2 teaspoon vanilla extract
- Fresh berries or sliced fruit, for serving

Instructions:

1. In a bowl, whisk together chia seeds, almond milk, cocoa powder, honey or maple syrup, and vanilla extract until well combined.
2. Cover and refrigerate for at least 2 hours or overnight, stirring occasionally, until the mixture thickens into a pudding-like consistency.
3. Once the chia seed pudding is ready, spoon it into serving glasses or bowls.
4. Serve topped with fresh berries or sliced fruit for a delicious and indulgent treat.

Healthy Banana Ice Cream:

Ingredients:

- 4 ripe bananas, peeled and sliced

- 2 tablespoons almond butter or peanut butter
- 1 teaspoon vanilla extract
- Optional toppings: chopped nuts, dark chocolate chips, shredded coconut

Instructions:

1. Place sliced bananas in a single layer on a baking sheet lined with parchment paper.
2. Freeze bananas for at least 2 hours or until firm.
3. Once frozen, transfer bananas to a food processor.
4. Add almond butter or peanut butter and vanilla extract to the food processor.
5. Blend until smooth and creamy, scraping down the sides of the food processor as needed.
6. Serve immediately as soft-serve ice cream or transfer to a container and freeze for 1-2 hours for a firmer texture.
7. Serve healthy banana ice cream topped with chopped nuts, dark chocolate chips, or shredded coconut for added flavor and crunch.

CHAPTER EIGHT

Side Dishes That Complement Any Meal

Simple and Delicious Vegetable Side Dishes

Vegetable side dishes are not only nutritious but also versatile and flavorful. Here are some simple and delicious vegetable side dishes to complement any meal:

Roasted Garlic Parmesan Brussels Sprouts:

Ingredients:

- 1 pound Brussels sprouts, trimmed and halved
- 2 tablespoons olive oil
- 4 cloves garlic, minced
- 1/4 cup grated Parmesan cheese
- Salt and pepper to taste

Instructions:

1. Preheat the oven to 400°F (200°C). Line a baking sheet with parchment paper.
2. In a large bowl, toss Brussels sprouts with olive oil, minced garlic, grated Parmesan cheese, salt, and pepper until well coated.

3. Spread Brussels sprouts in a single layer on the prepared baking sheet.

4. Roast in the preheated oven for 20-25 minutes, tossing halfway through, until Brussels sprouts are tender and caramelized.

5. Serve hot as a flavorful and nutritious side dish.

Garlic Herb Roasted Carrots:

Ingredients:

- 1 pound carrots, peeled and sliced into sticks
- 2 tablespoons olive oil
- 3 cloves garlic, minced
- 1 teaspoon dried thyme
- 1 teaspoon dried rosemary
- Salt and pepper to taste
- Fresh parsley, chopped, for garnish

Instructions:

1. Preheat the oven to 400°F (200°C). Line a baking sheet with parchment paper.

2. In a large bowl, toss carrot sticks with olive oil, minced garlic, dried thyme, dried rosemary, salt, and pepper until well coated.

3. Spread carrots in a single layer on the prepared baking sheet.

4. Roast in the preheated oven for 20-25 minutes, tossing halfway through, until carrots are tender and caramelized.

5. Garnish with chopped fresh parsley before serving.

Sauteed Garlic Green Beans:

Ingredients:

- 1 pound green beans, trimmed
- 2 tablespoons olive oil
- 3 cloves garlic, minced
- Salt and pepper to taste
- Lemon wedges, for serving

Instructions:

1. Heat olive oil in a large skillet over medium heat.

2. Add minced garlic to the skillet and cook until fragrant, about 1 minute.

3. Add green beans to the skillet and sauté for 5-7 minutes until tender-crisp.

4. Season with salt and pepper to taste.

5. Transfer green beans to a serving dish and squeeze lemon wedges over the top before serving.

Whole Grain and Legume-Based Sides for Balanced Nutrition

Incorporating whole grains and legumes into your side dishes adds fiber, protein, and essential nutrients to your meals. Here are some options for balanced nutrition:

Quinoa Pilaf with Mixed Vegetables:

Ingredients:

- 1 cup quinoa, rinsed
- 2 cups vegetable broth
- 1 tablespoon olive oil
- 1 onion, chopped
- 2 cloves garlic, minced
- 1 cup mixed vegetables (such as bell peppers, carrots, peas)
- Salt and pepper to taste
- Chopped fresh herbs (such as parsley or cilantro), for garnish

Instructions:

1. In a saucepan, combine quinoa and vegetable broth. Bring to a boil.
2. Reduce heat, cover, and simmer for 15-20 minutes until quinoa is cooked and liquid is absorbed.
3. In a separate skillet, heat olive oil over medium heat.
4. Add chopped onion and minced garlic to the skillet. Cook until softened, about 2-3 minutes.
5. Add mixed vegetables to the skillet and sauté until tender.
6. Stir cooked vegetables into the cooked quinoa. Season with salt and pepper to taste.
7. Garnish with chopped fresh herbs before serving.

Spiced Lentil and Brown Rice Pilaf:

Ingredients:

- 1 cup brown rice
- 1/2 cup dried green or brown lentils
- 3 cups vegetable broth
- 1 tablespoon olive oil
- 1 onion, chopped
- 2 cloves garlic, minced

- 1 teaspoon ground cumin
- 1/2 teaspoon ground coriander
- 1/2 teaspoon paprika
- Salt and pepper to taste
- Chopped fresh cilantro, for garnish

Instructions:

1. In a saucepan, combine brown rice, dried lentils, and vegetable broth. Bring to a boil.
2. Reduce heat, cover, and simmer for 35-40 minutes until rice and lentils are tender and liquid is absorbed.
3. In a separate skillet, heat olive oil over medium heat.
4. Add chopped onion and minced garlic to the skillet. Cook until softened, about 2-3 minutes.
5. Stir in ground cumin, ground coriander, and paprika. Cook for an additional minute until fragrant.
6. Stir cooked spiced onion mixture into the cooked rice and lentils. Season with salt and pepper to taste.
7. Garnish with chopped fresh cilantro before serving.

Mediterranean Chickpea Salad:

Ingredients:

- 2 cups cooked chickpeas (canned or cooked from dried)
- 1 cucumber, diced
- 1 bell pepper, diced
- 1/4 red onion, thinly sliced
- 1/4 cup Kalamata olives, pitted and sliced
- 2 tablespoons olive oil
- 1 tablespoon red wine vinegar
- 1 teaspoon dried oregano
- Salt and pepper to taste
- Crumbled feta cheese (optional)
- Chopped fresh parsley, for garnish

Instructions:

1. In a large bowl, combine cooked chickpeas, diced cucumber, diced bell pepper, thinly sliced red onion, and sliced Kalamata olives.
2. In a small bowl, whisk together olive oil, red wine vinegar, dried oregano, salt, and pepper to make the dressing.
3. Pour the dressing over the chickpea salad and toss to coat evenly.

4. If desired, sprinkle crumbled feta cheese over the salad.

5. Garnish with chopped fresh parsley before serving.

8.3 Creative Ways to Add Flavor to Your Side Dishes

Enhance the flavor of your side dishes with creative ingredient combinations and cooking techniques. Here are some ideas to try:

Herb-Roasted Potatoes with Garlic Aioli:

Ingredients:

- 1 pound baby potatoes, halved
- 2 tablespoons olive oil
- 2 cloves garlic, minced
- 1 teaspoon dried rosemary
- 1 teaspoon dried thyme
- Salt and pepper to taste
- Fresh parsley, chopped, for garnish

Instructions:

1. Preheat the oven to 400°F (200°C). Line a baking sheet with parchment paper.

2. In a bowl, toss halved baby potatoes with olive oil, minced garlic, dried rosemary, dried thyme, salt, and pepper until well coated.

3. Spread potatoes in a single layer on the prepared baking sheet.

4. Roast in the preheated oven for 25-30 minutes, tossing halfway through, until potatoes are golden and crispy.

5. Garnish with chopped fresh parsley before serving. Serve with garlic aioli for dipping.

Sesame Ginger Glazed Carrots:

Ingredients:

- 1 pound carrots, peeled and sliced into sticks
- 2 tablespoons sesame oil
- 2 tablespoons soy sauce (or tamari for gluten-free option)
- 1 tablespoon honey or maple syrup
- 1 teaspoon grated ginger
- 1 tablespoon sesame seeds
- Fresh cilantro, chopped, for garnish

Instructions:

1. In a skillet, heat sesame oil over medium heat.

2. Add sliced carrots to the skillet and sauté for 5-7 minutes until tender-crisp.

3. In a small bowl, whisk together soy sauce, honey or maple syrup, and grated ginger.

4. Pour the sauce over the carrots in the skillet and toss to coat evenly.

5. Cook for an additional 2-3 minutes until the sauce thickens and coats the carrots.

6. Sprinkle sesame seeds over the glazed carrots.

7. Garnish with chopped fresh cilantro before serving.

Balsamic Roasted Asparagus with Parmesan:

Ingredients:

- 1 pound asparagus, trimmed
- 2 tablespoons olive oil
- 2 tablespoons balsamic vinegar
- 2 cloves garlic, minced
- Salt and pepper to taste
- 1/4 cup grated Parmesan cheese
- Lemon wedges, for serving

Instructions:

1. Preheat the oven to 400°F (200°C). Line a baking sheet with parchment paper.

2. In a bowl, toss trimmed asparagus with olive oil, balsamic vinegar, minced garlic, salt, and pepper until well coated.

3. Spread asparagus in a single layer on the prepared baking sheet.

4. Roast in the preheated oven for 12-15 minutes until asparagus is tender and slightly caramelized.

5. Sprinkle grated Parmesan cheese over the roasted asparagus.

6. Serve hot with lemon wedges for squeezing over the top.

CHAPTER NINE

Eating Out and Socializing with Diabetes

Strategies for Making Healthy Choices When Dining Out

Eating out can present challenges for individuals managing diabetes, but with the right strategies, it's possible to make healthy choices while enjoying restaurant meals:

Research Menus in Advance: Before dining out, take some time to look up the menu online. Many restaurants now provide nutritional information alongside their menu items, which can help you make informed choices.

Choose Grilled or Baked Options: Opt for grilled, baked, or broiled dishes instead of fried ones. These cooking methods often use less added fat, reducing the overall calorie and carbohydrate content of the meal.

Request Modifications: Don't be afraid to ask for modifications to dishes to better suit your dietary needs. Requesting sauces and dressings on the side, asking for steamed vegetables instead of fries, or substituting whole grains for refined grains are all ways to make your meal healthier.

Watch Portion Sizes: Restaurant portions tend to be larger than what you might serve yourself at home. Consider sharing an entree with a dining companion or asking for a to-go box at the beginning of the meal to portion out half of your meal for later.

Be Mindful of Hidden Sugars: Keep an eye out for hidden sugars in sauces, dressings, and condiments. Opt for dishes that are prepared with minimal added sugars or ask if sugar-free options are available.

Limit Alcohol Intake: Alcoholic beverages can raise blood sugar levels and add empty calories to your meal. If you choose to drink alcohol, do so in moderation and opt for lower-carbohydrate options like light beer, dry wine, or spirits mixed with soda water.

Tips for Navigating Social Events and Special Occasions

Social events and special occasions often revolve around food, which can make managing diabetes challenging. Here are some tips for navigating these situations while still enjoying yourself:

Plan Ahead: If you know you'll be attending a social event or special occasion, plan your meals and snacks for the rest of the day accordingly. This can help you balance your blood sugar levels and prevent overindulging later on.

Bring a Dish: Offer to bring a diabetes-friendly dish to share at gatherings. This ensures that you'll have at least one option that aligns with your dietary needs, and others may appreciate the healthier option as well.

Focus on Socializing: Shift the focus away from food by engaging in conversations, participating in activities, or simply enjoying the company of others. Remember that social events are about more than just eating.

Practice Portion Control: When faced with a buffet or a spread of appetizers, practice portion control by using a smaller plate, filling half your plate with vegetables, and limiting high-carbohydrate options.

Stay Hydrated: Drink plenty of water throughout the event to stay hydrated and help control your appetite. Sometimes thirst can be mistaken for hunger, leading to overeating.

Be Prepared for Questions: Be prepared to answer questions about your dietary choices and diabetes management. Educate others about your needs and preferences in a positive and informative manner.

9.3 How to Communicate Your Dietary Needs Effectively

Communicating your dietary needs effectively is crucial when dining out or attending social events. Here are some tips for effectively communicating your needs:

Be Clear and Specific: Clearly communicate your dietary restrictions, preferences, and needs to restaurant staff or hosts. Provide specific instructions or ask questions to ensure that your needs are understood.

Use Positive Language: Frame your dietary requests in a positive light. Instead of saying what you can't eat, focus on what you can eat or what modifications would make a dish suitable for you.

Ask Questions: Don't hesitate to ask questions about menu items, ingredients, or how dishes are prepared. This can help you make informed choices and avoid any surprises.

Express Appreciation: Express gratitude to restaurant staff or hosts for accommodating your dietary needs. A simple thank you goes a long way in fostering positive communication.

Be Flexible: Be open to suggestions or alternatives if your specific requests cannot be accommodated. Flexibility can help ensure a more enjoyable dining experience for everyone involved.

Follow Up: If you have any concerns or questions about the food served, don't hesitate to follow up with restaurant staff or hosts. Your feedback can help improve future dining experiences for yourself and others.

CHAPTER TEN

Meal Planning and Preparation Made Easy

Practical Tips for Meal Planning and Grocery Shopping

Meal planning and grocery shopping are essential steps in maintaining a healthy diet, especially for individuals managing diabetes. Here are some practical tips to make meal planning and grocery shopping easier:

Set Aside Time for Planning: Designate a specific time each week to plan your meals and create a shopping list. This could be a weekend morning or whichever day works best for you.

Plan Balanced Meals: Focus on creating balanced meals that include a variety of foods from different food groups, such as lean proteins, whole grains, healthy fats, and plenty of fruits and vegetables. Aim for a mix of colors and textures to ensure you're getting a wide range of nutrients.

Take Inventory: Before making your shopping list, take inventory of what you already have in your pantry, refrigerator, and freezer. This helps prevent overbuying and reduces food waste.

Make a Detailed Shopping List: Based on your planned meals and inventory, create a detailed shopping list organized by food categories (e.g., produce, dairy, proteins). Stick to your list to avoid impulse purchases.

Shop the Perimeter of the Store: Focus on purchasing fresh produce, lean proteins, dairy products, and whole grains, which are typically located around the perimeter of the grocery store. This helps you avoid processed and unhealthy foods found in the center aisles.

Read Nutrition Labels: When selecting packaged foods, read nutrition labels carefully to check for added sugars, sodium, and unhealthy fats. Choose items with lower amounts of these ingredients and prioritize whole, minimally processed foods.

Buy in Bulk: For staple items that you use regularly (e.g., grains, beans, frozen vegetables), consider buying in bulk to save money and reduce the frequency of shopping trips.

Plan for Leftovers: Intentionally cook extra portions to have leftovers for future meals. This can save time and effort on busy days when you don't feel like cooking from scratch.

Use Technology: Take advantage of meal planning apps or websites that offer customizable recipes, grocery lists, and nutritional information. These tools can streamline the planning process and help you stay organized.

Stay Flexible: Be flexible with your meal plan and shopping list. If certain ingredients are unavailable or on sale, be willing to make substitutions or adjustments to your plan.

Batch Cooking and Freezing Meals for Convenience

Batch cooking and freezing meals in advance can save time and make healthy eating more convenient, especially for busy individuals managing diabetes. Here are some strategies to consider:

Choose Freezer-Friendly Recipes: Select recipes that freeze well and maintain their quality when reheated, such as soups, stews, casseroles, and chili.

Invest in Freezer-Friendly Containers: Use freezer-safe containers or resealable bags to portion and store meals. Label containers with the contents and date of preparation for easy identification.

Cook in Batches: Set aside a few hours on a weekend or whenever you have time to cook in larger batches. Prepare multiple servings of your favorite recipes to freeze for later use.

Portion Meals Before Freezing: Divide batch-cooked meals into individual or family-sized portions before freezing. This makes it easier to thaw and reheat only what you need for a single meal.

Flash Freeze Ingredients: For recipes that call for individually frozen ingredients (e.g., berries, vegetables), spread them out on a baking sheet and place them in the freezer until frozen solid. Then transfer them to freezer bags for long-term storage.

Keep an Inventory: Maintain a freezer inventory list to keep track of what meals you have on hand and when they were prepared. Rotate older items to the front of the freezer to ensure nothing goes to waste.

Thaw Safely: Plan ahead and thaw frozen meals safely in the refrigerator overnight or use the defrost setting on your microwave. Avoid thawing at room temperature to prevent bacterial growth.

Reheat Properly: When reheating frozen meals, use appropriate methods such as the stovetop, oven, or microwave. Ensure that food reaches a safe internal temperature before serving.

Experiment with New Recipes: Use batch cooking as an opportunity to experiment with new recipes or variations of your favorite dishes. This keeps mealtime interesting and prevents boredom with your meal rotation.

Strategies for Portion Control and Balanced Eating

Portion control is key to managing blood sugar levels and maintaining a healthy weight. Here are some strategies to help you control portions and eat balanced meals:

Use Smaller Plates: Opt for smaller plates and bowls to visually trick yourself into thinking you're eating more than you actually are. This can help prevent overeating.

Fill Half Your Plate with Vegetables: Make vegetables the star of your meals by filling half your plate with non-starchy vegetables like leafy greens, broccoli, and bell peppers. This adds volume and fiber to your meal without adding excess calories or carbohydrates.

Practice the Plate Method: Follow the plate method by dividing your plate into sections: half for vegetables, a quarter for lean protein, and a quarter for whole grains or starchy vegetables. This helps ensure a balanced and portion-controlled meal.

Measure Portions: Use measuring cups, spoons, or a kitchen scale to portion out serving sizes of foods, especially high-calorie or high-carbohydrate items like grains, nuts, and dried fruits.

Be Mindful of Snacking: Snack mindfully by portioning out snacks into small bowls or containers instead of eating directly from the package. This helps prevent mindless eating and encourages portion control.

Slow Down and Chew Thoroughly: Eat slowly and chew your food thoroughly to give your body time to register feelings of fullness. This can prevent overeating and promote better digestion.

Listen to Your Hunger Cues: Pay attention to your body's hunger and fullness signals. Eat when you're hungry and stop when you're satisfied, rather than eating until you're overly full.

Practice Moderation with Treats: Enjoy your favorite treats in moderation, but be mindful of portion sizes and frequency. Consider sharing desserts or indulging in smaller portions to satisfy your cravings without overindulging.

Stay Hydrated: Drink water throughout the day to stay hydrated and help regulate appetite. Sometimes thirst can be mistaken for hunger, leading to overeating.

CHAPTER 12
31 DAY MEAL PLAN

Week 1:

Day 1:

- Breakfast: Greek yogurt with mixed berries and a sprinkle of chia seeds
- Snack: Carrot sticks with hummus
- Lunch: Turkey and avocado wrap with whole grain tortilla
- Snack: Handful of almonds
- Dinner: Baked salmon with roasted vegetables

Day 2:

- Breakfast: Oatmeal with sliced bananas and a drizzle of honey
- Snack: Apple slices with almond butter
- Lunch: Quinoa salad with mixed greens, cherry tomatoes, and feta cheese
- Snack: Celery sticks with cream cheese
- Dinner: Grilled chicken breast with steamed broccoli

Day 3:

- Breakfast: Scrambled eggs with spinach and tomatoes
- Snack: Greek yogurt with a handful of walnuts
- Lunch: Tuna salad lettuce wraps with cucumber slices
- Snack: Cherry tomatoes with mozzarella cheese
- Dinner: Beef stir-fry with bell peppers and brown rice

Day 4:

- Breakfast: Whole grain toast with avocado slices and a boiled egg
- Snack: Cottage cheese with pineapple chunks
- Lunch: Veggie omelette with a side salad
- Snack: Mixed nuts
- Dinner: Baked cod with quinoa and roasted asparagus

Day 5:

- Breakfast: Smoothie made with spinach, banana, and unsweetened almond milk
- Snack: Apple slices with peanut butter
- Lunch: Grilled shrimp skewers with zucchini noodles and marinara sauce
- Snack: Carrot sticks with hummus

- Dinner: Turkey chili with a side of whole grain crackers

Day 6:

- Breakfast: Cottage cheese with sliced peaches and a sprinkle of cinnamon
- Snack: Greek yogurt with mixed berries
- Lunch: Turkey and cheese roll-ups with cucumber slices
- Snack: Handful of almonds
- Dinner: Stir-fried tofu with mixed vegetables and brown rice

Day 7:

- Breakfast: Whole grain cereal with low-fat milk and a handful of berries
- Snack: Carrot sticks with hummus
- Lunch: Chicken Caesar salad with a light dressing
- Snack: Cherry tomatoes with mozzarella cheese
- Dinner: Baked chicken thighs with roasted Brussels sprouts

Week 2:

Day 8:

- Breakfast: Scrambled eggs with diced bell peppers and onions

- Snack: Greek yogurt with a handful of walnuts
- Lunch: Veggie wrap with hummus and sliced bell peppers
- Snack: Celery sticks with cream cheese
- Dinner: Baked salmon with quinoa and roasted vegetables

Day 9:

- Breakfast: Oatmeal with sliced apples and a sprinkle of cinnamon
- Snack: Apple slices with almond butter
- Lunch: Tuna salad lettuce wraps with avocado
- Snack: Mixed nuts
- Dinner: Beef stir-fry with broccoli and brown rice

Day 10:

- Breakfast: Whole grain toast with avocado slices and a boiled egg
- Snack: Cottage cheese with pineapple chunks
- Lunch: Quinoa salad with black beans, corn, and cherry tomatoes
- Snack: Carrot sticks with hummus
- Dinner: Grilled chicken breast with steamed asparagus

Day 11:

- Breakfast: Greek yogurt with mixed berries and a sprinkle of chia seeds
- Snack: Greek yogurt with a handful of walnuts
- Lunch: Turkey and avocado wrap with lettuce and tomato
- Snack: Celery sticks with cream cheese
- Dinner: Baked cod with quinoa and roasted vegetables

Day 12:

- Breakfast: Smoothie made with spinach, banana, and unsweetened almond milk
- Snack: Apple slices with almond butter
- Lunch: Chicken Caesar salad with a light dressing
- Snack: Mixed nuts
- Dinner: Stir-fried tofu with mixed vegetables and brown rice

Day 13:

- Breakfast: Cottage cheese with sliced peaches and a sprinkle of cinnamon
- Snack: Greek yogurt with a handful of walnuts
- Lunch: Veggie omelette with a side salad

- Snack: Celery sticks with cream cheese
- Dinner: Baked chicken thighs with roasted Brussels sprouts

Day 14:

- Breakfast: Whole grain cereal with low-fat milk and a handful of berries
- Snack: Greek yogurt with a handful of walnuts
- Lunch: Turkey and cheese roll-ups with cucumber slices
- Snack: Mixed nuts
- Dinner: Baked salmon with quinoa and roasted vegetables

Week 3:

Day 15:

- Breakfast: Scrambled eggs with diced bell peppers and onions
- Snack: Apple slices with almond butter
- Lunch: Grilled shrimp skewers with zucchini noodles and marinara sauce
- Snack: Carrot sticks with hummus
- Dinner: Beef stir-fry with broccoli and brown rice

Day 16:

- Breakfast: Oatmeal with sliced bananas and a drizzle of honey
- Snack: Greek yogurt with a handful of walnuts
- Lunch: Turkey and avocado wrap with lettuce and tomato
- Snack: Celery sticks with cream cheese
- Dinner: Baked chicken breast with quinoa and roasted vegetables

Day 17:

- Breakfast: Whole grain toast with avocado slices and a boiled egg
- Snack: Cottage cheese with pineapple chunks
- Lunch: Quinoa salad with black beans, corn, and cherry tomatoes
- Snack: Carrot sticks with hummus
- Dinner: Grilled salmon with steamed asparagus

Day 18:

- Breakfast: Greek yogurt with mixed berries and a sprinkle of chia seeds
- Snack: Greek yogurt with a handful of walnuts
- Lunch: Veggie wrap with hummus and sliced bell peppers

- Snack: Mixed nuts
- Dinner: Beef stir-fry with broccoli and brown rice

Day 19:

- Breakfast: Smoothie made with spinach, banana, and unsweetened almond milk
- Snack: Apple slices with almond butter
- Lunch: Chicken Caesar salad with a light dressing
- Snack: Celery sticks with cream cheese
- Dinner: Baked cod with quinoa and roasted vegetables

Day 20:

- Breakfast: Cottage cheese with sliced peaches and a sprinkle of cinnamon
- Snack: Greek yogurt with a handful of walnuts
- Lunch: Turkey and cheese roll-ups with cucumber slices
- Snack: Carrot sticks with hummus
- Dinner: Stir-fried tofu with mixed vegetables and brown rice

Day 21:

- Breakfast: Whole grain cereal with low-fat milk and a handful of berries

- Snack: Greek yogurt with a handful of walnuts
- Lunch: Grilled shrimp skewers with zucchini noodles and marinara sauce
- Snack: Mixed nuts
- Dinner: Baked chicken thighs with roasted Brussels sprouts

Week 4:

Day 22:

- Breakfast: Scrambled eggs with diced bell peppers and onions
- Snack: Apple slices with almond butter
- Lunch: Turkey and avocado wrap with lettuce and tomato
- Snack: Celery sticks with cream cheese
- Dinner: Baked salmon with quinoa and roasted vegetables

Day 23:

- Breakfast: Oatmeal with sliced bananas and a drizzle of honey
- Snack: Greek yogurt with a handful of walnuts
- Lunch: Quinoa salad with black beans, corn, and cherry tomatoes

- Snack: Carrot sticks with hummus
- Dinner: Beef stir-fry with broccoli and brown rice

Day 24:

- Breakfast: Whole grain toast with avocado slices and a boiled egg
- Snack: Cottage cheese with pineapple chunks
- Lunch: Veggie wrap with hummus and sliced bell peppers
- Snack: Mixed nuts
- Dinner: Grilled chicken breast with steamed asparagus

Day 25:

- Breakfast: Greek yogurt with mixed berries and a sprinkle of chia seeds
- Snack: Apple slices with almond butter
- Lunch: Chicken Caesar salad with a light dressing
- Snack: Celery sticks with cream cheese
- Dinner: Baked cod with quinoa and roasted vegetables

Day 26:

- Breakfast: Smoothie made with spinach, banana, and unsweetened almond milk

- Snack: Greek yogurt with a handful of walnuts
- Lunch: Turkey and cheese roll-ups with cucumber slices
- Snack: Carrot sticks with hummus
- Dinner: Stir-fried tofu with mixed vegetables and brown rice

Day 27:

- Breakfast: Cottage cheese with sliced peaches and a sprinkle of cinnamon
- Snack: Apple slices with almond butter
- Lunch: Grilled shrimp skewers with zucchini noodles and marinara sauce
- Snack: Celery sticks with cream cheese
- Dinner: Beef stir-fry with broccoli and brown rice

Day 28:

- Breakfast: Whole grain cereal with low-fat milk and a handful of berries
- Snack: Greek yogurt with a handful of walnuts
- Lunch: Turkey and avocado wrap with lettuce and tomato
- Snack: Mixed nuts
- Dinner: Baked salmon with quinoa and roasted vegetables

Day 29:

- Breakfast: Scrambled eggs with diced bell peppers and onions
- Snack: Apple slices with almond butter
- Lunch: Quinoa salad with black beans, corn, and cherry tomatoes
- Snack: Carrot sticks with hummus
- Dinner: Grilled chicken breast with steamed asparagus

Day 30:

- Breakfast: Oatmeal with sliced bananas and a drizzle of honey
- Snack: Greek yogurt with a handful of walnuts
- Lunch: Chicken Caesar salad with a light dressing
- Snack: Celery sticks with cream cheese
- Dinner: Baked cod with quinoa and roasted vegetables

Day 31:

- Breakfast: Greek yogurt with mixed berries and a sprinkle of chia seeds
- Snack: Apple slices with almond butter

- Lunch: Turkey and cheese roll-ups with cucumber slices
- Snack: Carrot sticks with hummus
- Dinner: Beef stir-fry with broccoli and brown rice

THE END

www.ingramcontent.com/pod-product-compliance
Lightning Source LLC
Chambersburg PA
CBHW082340220526
45470CB00008B/2586